D1712479

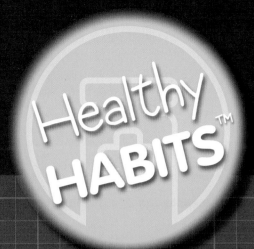

Healthy HABITS ™

Vitamins and Minerals

Getting the Nutrients Your Body Needs

Stephanie Watson

rosen publishing's
rosen central®

Published in 2011 by The Rosen Publishing Group, Inc.
29 East 21st Street, New York, NY 10010

First Edition

Library of Congress Cataloging-in-Publication Data

Watson, Stephanie, 1969–
Vitamins and minerals: getting the nutrients your body needs / Stephanie Watson.—1st ed.
    p. cm.—(Healthy habits)
Includes bibliographical references and index.
ISBN 978-1-4358-9443-3 (library binding)
ISBN 978-1-4488-0613-3 (pbk)
ISBN 978-1-4488-0617-1 (6-pack)
1. Vitamins in human nutrition—Juvenile literature. 2. Minerals in human nutrition—Juvenile literature. I. Title.
QP771.W38 2011
612.3'99—dc22

2009054121

Manufactured in Malaysia

CPSIA Compliance Information: Batch #S10YA: For further information, contact Rosen Publishing, New York, New York, at 1-800-237-9932.

CONTENTS

Introduction..............................4

CHAPTER 1 Which Vitamins Does the Body Need? .. 7

CHAPTER 2 Minerals and Other Essential

Ingredients of a Healthy Diet...........19

CHAPTER 3 Dangers of Skimping on

Vitamins and Minerals 27

CHAPTER 4 Building a Healthy, Balanced Diet 42

Glossary..................................53

For More Information....................55

For Further Reading 58

Bibliography.............................60

Index..................................62

Cars need fuel to run. When a car runs out of gas, it stops going. Humans also need fuel (in their case, food) to keep running. If people don't eat, they can't survive.

Both cars and humans not only need fuel, but also they need the right kind of fuel to run at their best. Put the wrong grade of gasoline in a car's tank, and it won't drive right. Eat a steady diet of fast-food burgers and French fries, and the body won't function as well as it should.

The human body is designed to work most efficiently when it is supplied with a steady combination of different vitamins, minerals, and other nutrients. These healthy ingredients keep cells and organs functioning properly, enable the body to grow and develop, and help the immune system fight off illness.

Thirteen vitamins are absolutely essential for human survival: vitamins A, D, E, K, C, and eight different B vitamins. The body needs these vitamins in relatively large quantities. Certain minerals, such as calcium, magnesium, and potassium, are also necessary to keep the body running in top form. Other minerals, including iron, zinc, and copper, are only needed in small amounts. They are called trace minerals.

The human body is able to produce small amounts of certain vitamins, such as vitamins D and K. However, most of the vitamins and minerals that the body needs come from foods. Plants and animals are naturally rich in a variety of nutrients. They absorb these nutrients from the earth and water. When people eat plants and animals, their bodies take in the nutrients.

Although each person's nutritional needs are different, every-one must eat a balanced diet to stay healthy. Snacks such as

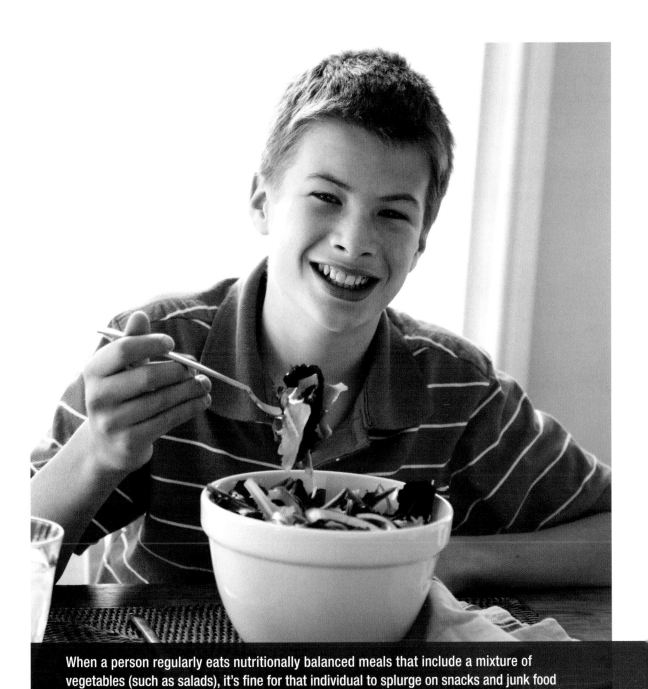

When a person regularly eats nutritionally balanced meals that include a mixture of vegetables (such as salads), it's fine for that individual to splurge on snacks and junk food once in a while.

potato chips, cookies, and sodas are unhealthy because they contain almost no vitamins and minerals, and they are full of sugar, salt, fat, and calories. Eating these junk foods once in a while is OK, but filling up on them regularly leaves less room for healthy foods. Eating a lot of junk food can also lead to obesity and diseases related to obesity, such as heart disease and diabetes.

When people do not get enough nutrients from their diet, they can end up with a vitamin or mineral deficiency. This lack of nutrients can lead to disease. For example, not getting enough vitamin D can cause weak, brittle bones that break easily, and it can increase the risk for heart disease and certain types of cancer later in life. Despite these risks, 70 percent of young people in the United States do not get enough vitamin D in their diet, according to a study in the August 2009 issue of *Pediatrics*.

The best way to stay healthy and prevent disease is to get the right mix of vitamins and minerals in the diet by eating a variety of fruits, vegetables, whole grains, dairy products, lean meats, fish, and poultry. Adding in other healthy habits, such as getting adequate sleep and exercising regularly, will ensure that the body stays in top shape for many years to come.

Chapter 1

Which Vitamins Does the Body Need?

Vitamins and minerals are essential to the human body because these nutrients carry out a variety of chemical reactions. These reactions drive just about every function the body requires to stay alive and functioning properly.

The body absolutely can't live without thirteen vitamins: A, D, E, K, C, and eight different B vitamins. Before learning about these important vitamins, it's helpful to understand the difference between the two types of vitamins: water-soluble and fat-soluble.

Types of Vitamins

Vitamins C and the B complex vitamins are examples of water-soluble vitamins. The body easily absorbs these vitamins through the bloodstream and uses them right away. Because water-soluble vitamins are not stored in the body, people must take them every day to get the amount they need. When someone takes more water-soluble vitamins than the body requires, the kidneys simply filter the excess into the urine.

Fat-soluble vitamins A, D, E, and K are stored in the liver and fat tissues. They stay there until the body needs them. Because fat-soluble

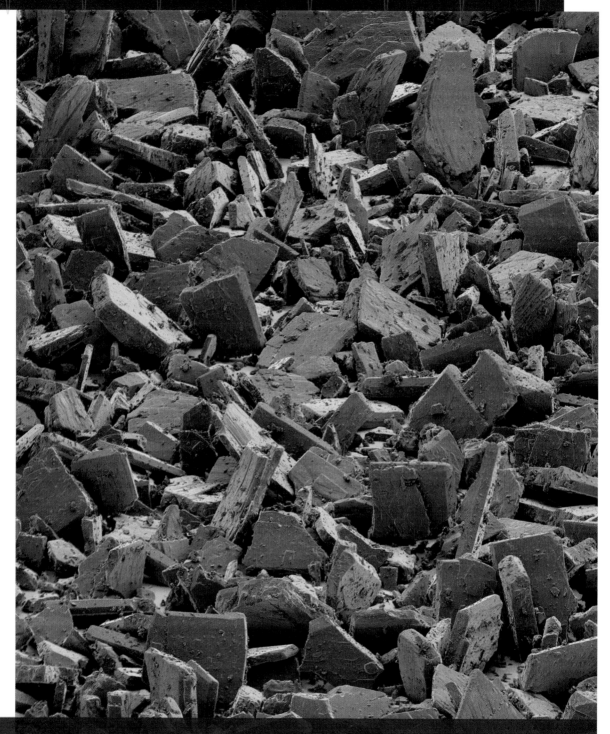

These magnified crystals are vitamin C, a water-soluble vitamin. Vitamin C is an antioxidant, which helps protect the body's cells from damage that could lead to disease.

vitamins remain in the body for long periods of time, taking large amounts of these vitamins can be dangerous.

Vitamin A

There is a reason why many mothers urge their children to eat their carrots. Mom was right—carrots do help keep vision sharp. They're packed with vitamin A, a water-soluble vitamin that is also important for growth, healthy skin, reproduction, and cell division. Spinach, liver, and kale are other excellent sources of this vitamin. Vitamin A is involved in the production of white blood cells—the army of immune system cells that helps the body fight off infections.

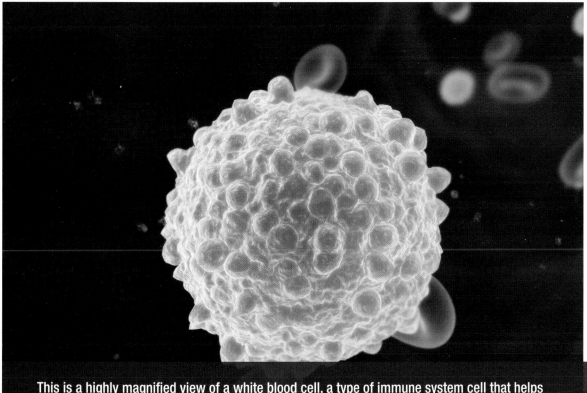

This is a highly magnified view of a white blood cell, a type of immune system cell that helps defend the body against invaders called pathogens. Pathogens can cause disease.

Vitamin A claimed its place at the head of the alphabet because it was the first vitamin to be officially named. This vitamin comes in different forms. Carotenoids are the form of vitamin A found in foods. They are the pigments that give fruits and vegetables their brilliant red, yellow, and orange colors. Alpha- and beta-carotenoids are anti-oxidants. When the body is exposed to chemicals, pollution, smoke, and other harmful substances in the environment, it produces molecules called free radicals, which can damage cells and lead to cancer and other diseases. Antioxidants are substances that protect the body from damage caused by free radicals.

The body must convert carotenoids to a form called retinol to use them. Enzymes in the gastrointestinal tract help convert the carotenoids into active vitamin A. Although more than five hundred different carotenoids exist, fewer than 10 percent can be made into active vitamin A in the body. Of all the carotenoids, beta-carotene is the one the body turns into vitamin A most effectively.

Vitamin C

In the late 1920s, Hungarian biochemist Albert Szent-Györgyi discovered ascorbic acid, or vitamin C, as it is better known. Even as far back as the time of ancient Egypt, people understood that eating citrus fruits (which are high in vitamin C) could help promote healthy gums and general good health.

Vitamin C is an antioxidant that has a number of important functions. It helps the body protect itself against infections, which is why many people drink a lot of extra orange juice when they feel a cold coming on. Although vitamin C won't prevent colds and other viral infections, it can make them shorter and less severe, according to a 2007 study published in *American Family Physician*. When taken on a regular basis, vitamin C may also help protect against the fatty buildup in the arteries that can lead to a heart attack or stroke. It also improves the absorption of iron (an important mineral) from foods and supplements.

Linus Pauling, the Father of Vitamin C

Probably no one in history was a bigger fan of vitamin C than Nobel Prize–winning chemist Linus Pauling. In 1970, he wrote a book called *Vitamin C and the Common Cold*. Pauling claimed that taking big doses (megadoses) of vitamin C could not only ward off the common cold, but also prevent cancer. The book was very controversial, and many doctors did not agree with Pauling's theories.

Pauling recommended that people take at least 3 grams of vitamin C per day. For reference, the recommended daily dietary intake of vitamin C for adults is 60 milligrams. He himself took several grams of the vitamin every day, and he lived to be ninety-three years old.

Vitamin D

Vitamin D is sometimes called the "sunshine vitamin" because the body produces it when ultraviolet light from the sun strikes the skin. The body can produce 400 international units (IU) of vitamin D after just twenty minutes out in the sun with the skin exposed (the recommended daily intake of vitamin D for teens is 200 IU). Before using the vitamin D it absorbs from the sun, the body must convert it into an active form in the liver and kidneys. Some vitamin D also comes into the body from foods like milk and other dairy products, such as cheese. People who live in northern climates, those with very dark skin (which limits vitamin D absorption), and anyone who doesn't get out in the sun very often may need to take a supplement to ensure that they get the recommended amount of vitamin D each day. (However, people need to be careful about too much direct sun exposure, which can lead to premature aging and skin cancer.)

Vitamin D is calcium's partner in strengthening bones and teeth. It ensures that there is plenty of calcium in the bloodstream to supply the bones and teeth. Vitamin D keeps calcium levels in the blood high by increasing the absorption of calcium from the small

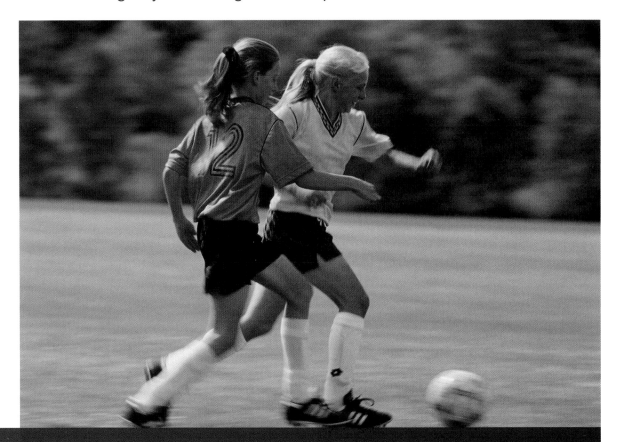

Vitamin D can help strengthen bones and protect them from fractures. Playing sports or getting other forms of exercise is another great way to keep the bones strong.

intestines, and by preventing too much calcium from being removed from the body in the urine. Vitamin D also helps regulate phosphorus levels. Phosphorus is important for healthy bones and teeth, and it helps the body store energy.

Vitamin E

Vitamin E is another example of an antioxidant—a substance that protects cells and tissues against the harmful effects of pollution, tobacco smoke, and ultraviolet radiation from the sun. This important vitamin, found in almonds, sunflower seeds, and some vegetable oils, helps keep the immune

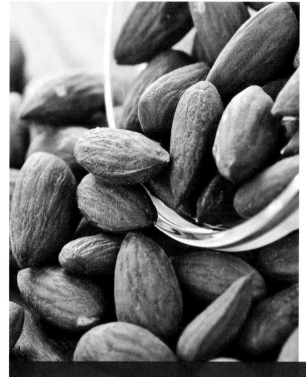

Almonds are an excellent source of vitamin E. One ounce (28.4 grams) of dry-roasted almonds contains 7.4 milligrams of vitamin E, which is 40 percent of the recommended daily value.

system healthy. It may also protect people from a wide variety of diseases, including heart disease, cancer, age-related macular degeneration (an eye disease that often affects elderly people), and Alzheimer's disease.

Vitamin K

The most important job of vitamin K is helping the blood to clot. Without this vitamin, which is found in olive and soybean oils and

DRIs: How Much People Need Each Day

Until the 1990s, the guideline for how much of each vitamin and mineral people needed to take every day was called the Recommended Daily Allowance (RDA). Today, that figure has been replaced by Dietary Reference Intakes (DRIs), a system of nutritional recommendations from the Institute of Medicine in Washington, D.C. The following are the daily DRIs for some of the most important vitamins and minerals.

Daily DRIs for Children Ages Nine to Thirteen:

Calcium	1,300 milligrams
Folate	300 micrograms
Iron	8 milligrams
Magnesium	240 milligrams
Potassium	4.5 grams
Vitamin A	600 micrograms
Vitamin B_6	1 milligrams
Vitamin B_{12}	1.8 milligrams
Vitamin C	45 milligrams
Vitamin D	5 micrograms
Vitamin E	11 milligrams
Vitamin K	60 micrograms

Daily DRIs for Teens Ages Fourteen to Eighteen:

Calcium	1,300 milligrams
Folate	400 micrograms
Iron	15 milligrams (females), 11 milligrams (males)
Magnesium	360 milligrams (females), 410 milligrams (males)
Potassium	4.7 grams
Vitamin A	700 micrograms (females), 900 micrograms (males)
Vitamin B_6	1.2 milligrams (females), 1.3 milligrams (males)
Vitamin B_{12}	2.4 milligrams
Vitamin C	65 milligrams (females), 75 milligrams (males)
Vitamin D	5 micrograms
Vitamin E	15 milligrams
Vitamin K	75 micrograms

[Source: Dietary Reference Intakes, Institute of Medicine, Washington, D.C., 2008]

in leafy green vegetables, a minor cut could lead to significant bleeding.

Vitamin K also regulates calcium levels in the blood and helps the bones and teeth use calcium to stay strong. It is believed to protect older adults from the disease called osteoporosis, which leads to brittle, easily breakable bones.

The B Vitamins

The B vitamin family has sixteen members in all, eight of which are essential to energy production, cell formation, and many other chemical reactions in the body. Enriched breads and cereals are excellent sources of these vitamins. Because B vitamins are water-soluble, people need to get them every day through food or supplements. The following is a quick introduction to some of the most important members of the B vitamin family:

B$_1$ (thiamine) is involved in energy metabolism. This vitamin ensures that the body is properly breaking down sugars for energy. It is also needed to

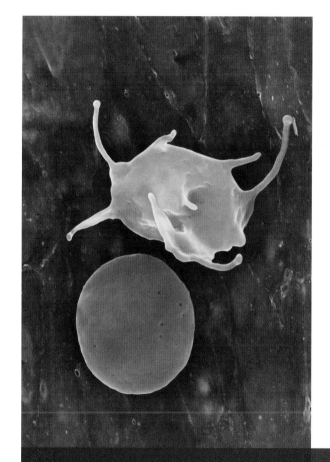

Vitamin K plays a very important role whenever people get minor cuts. It helps platelets in the blood form a clot, which prevents excess bleeding. Vitamin K can be found in green vegetables, such as broccoli, brussels sprouts, spinach, kale, collards, and turnip greens.

keep the brain and nervous system functioning as they should and to produce the chemicals that speed important messages from the brain to the rest of the body.

B$_2$ (riboflavin) helps the body turn proteins, carbohydrates, and fats from foods into energy. It strengthens the body's tissues to build healthy skin, hair, and nails. Vitamin B$_2$ also plays a role in growth, digestion, nervous system health, and vision.

B$_3$ (niacin) helps the body break down foods and use the protein, fats, and sugars inside for energy. It also keeps the nervous system and skin healthy. Vitamin B$_3$ is like the body's own natural cholesterol drug. It lowers levels of the unhealthy low-density lipoprotein (LDL) type of cholesterol, which can clog arteries and lead to heart disease. Furthermore, it raises levels of good high-density lipoprotein (HDL) cholesterol, which helps keep the arteries clear.

B$_5$ (pantothenic acid) is needed for energy metabolism. It helps cells break down fats and carbohydrates to release energy. Pantothenic acid also is involved in the production of hormones from the adrenal glands.

B$_6$ (pyridoxine) supports the nervous and immune systems, enables the body to produce hemoglobin (the substance in red blood cells that carries oxygen to the body's tissues), and keeps blood sugar levels constant. Vitamin B$_6$ is involved in dozens of different chemical reactions in the body, including the production of many different proteins.

B$_8$ (biotin) helps convert carbohydrates, fats, and proteins from foods into energy. Biotin also keeps hair, skin, and nails healthy.

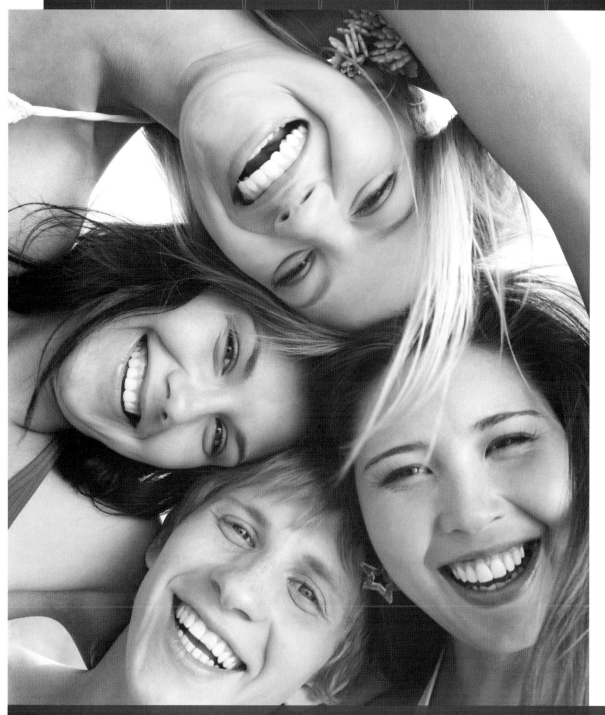

Vitamin B$_6$ is good for the body—inside and out. Also called pyridoxine, vitamin B$_6$, along with the other B vitamins, helps the body convert food into energy and keeps your skin, hair, and eyes healthy.

B₉ (folic acid) is involved in the production of deoxyribonucleic acid (DNA) and ribonucleic acid (RNA). DNA and RNA are the codes that direct the production of the proteins the body needs to work properly. Folic acid is also necessary for red blood cell formation. Researchers have discovered that folic acid can help reduce levels of homocysteine, an amino acid in the blood. At high levels, homocysteine can increase the risk of heart disease and excessive blood clotting.

Folic acid is especially important while a baby is developing in the mother's womb. When a mother takes folic acid every day during her pregnancy, it can help prevent birth defects such as spina bifida and cleft palate. Since 1998, the U.S. government has required manufacturers of breads, cereals, and other grain products to fortify their foods with folic acid. As a result, most Americans now get enough folic acid in their diet, and the number of birth defects due to low folic acid has declined.

B₁₂ (cyanocobalamin) helps produce DNA and maintains healthy nerve cells and red blood cells. Vitamin B₁₂ has so many different functions that not all of them are known yet. It may play a part in the production of chemical messengers in the brain called dopamine and serotonin, which affect mood and sleep patterns.

Vitamins aren't the only part of a healthy diet. The next chapter will take a look at the minerals that are also fundamental for a healthy body.

Chapter 2

Minerals and Other Essential Ingredients of a Healthy Diet

Many people think of minerals as rocks, such as diamonds or quartz, which are mined from the ground. Yet minerals are also an important part of the diet, and they are found in many of the foods people eat. This chapter covers some of the most important dietary minerals, along with a few other key components of a healthy diet.

Calcium

Most people immediately link calcium, which is found in milk, yogurt, and cheese, with bone health. It's true that the body needs calcium to maintain strong bones and teeth. In fact, about 99 percent of the calcium in the body is stored in the bones and teeth. This mineral is especially crucial to have during childhood and adolescence, when the bones are still growing. Vitamin D is calcium's partner in this process, helping the bones absorb calcium.

Providing bone strength is calcium's major job, but it also has other significant functions. Calcium helps transmit signals throughout the nervous system, widen or narrow blood vessels to let more or less blood flow through, and release the hormones that control many of the body's different activities.

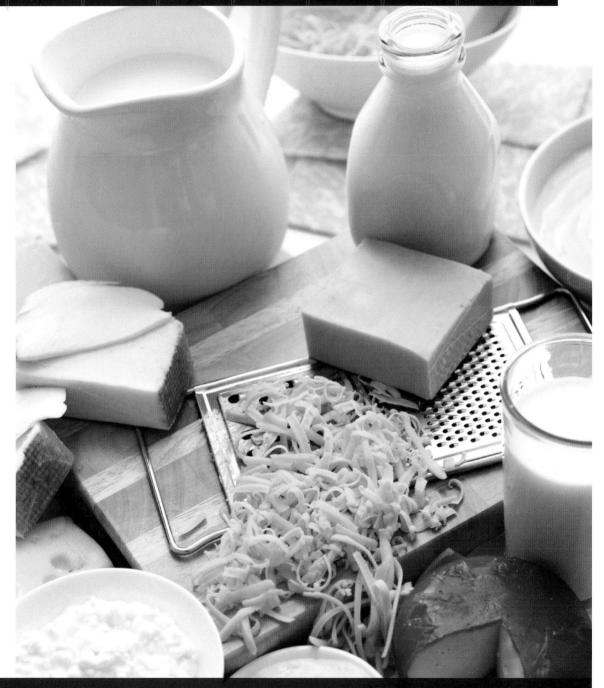

Milk, cheese, yogurt, and other dairy products are excellent sources of calcium, a mineral that helps build and maintain strong bones and teeth. If a person is unable to drink milk, that person can get calcium from drinking fortified soy milk or fruit juice.

Iron

Iron is one of the most plentiful minerals on Earth. It's essential for providing the body's tissues with the oxygen they need to work. Iron makes up an important part of hemoglobin, the protein that transports oxygen from the lungs to the body's tissues.

Two types of dietary iron exist: heme-bound and non-heme-bound. Heme-bound iron comes from hemoglobin. It is found in foods such as meat, fish, and poultry. Non-heme-bound iron is found in plants, such as lentils and beans. Most of the iron that enters the body through the diet is the non-heme form, although heme iron is easier for the body to absorb.

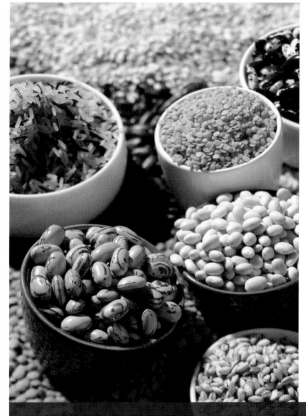

The non-heme-bound iron that is found in beans and lentils is harder for the body to absorb than the heme-bound iron that exists in meat and poultry. Therefore, many vegetarians need to take a supplement to get enough iron in their diets.

Potassium

Found mostly in the cells, potassium helps control blood pressure, regulates normal heart function, keeps the muscles contracting normally, and regulates the balance of fluid in the body's cells. Sweet potatoes and bananas are excellent food sources of this mineral. Potassium is an electrolyte, which means that it is involved in the body's electrical activities, supporting the movement of electrical signals across cell membranes.

Phosphorus

Phosphorus is one of the most abundant minerals in the human body, found in every one of the cells. Most phosphorus is stored in the bones and teeth, which it helps keep strong. Phosphorus is also needed to produce adenosine triphosphate (ATP), a molecule the body uses to store its energy. Some foods that are high in phosphorus include milk and other dairy products, peas, meat, and eggs.

Zinc

Many people take alternative cold remedies that contain zinc as an ingredient. Zinc, which is abundant in some meats and seafood, does help strengthen the immune system, and it can make colds shorter and less severe. Many of the body's systems rely on zinc, including the digestive system, senses (taste, vision, and smell), skin, and reproductive system. During childhood, zinc helps the body grow normally.

Iodine

The thyroid gland relies on iodine to make its hormones, thyroxine (T4), triiodothyronine (T3), and calcitonin. T4 and T3 help regulate the body's metabolism—the release of energy from foods eaten. Calcitonin regulates calcium levels in the body. Iodized table salt is an excellent source of this mineral.

Getting Enough Fiber in the Diet

Most people have heard that they need to get plenty of fiber in their diet. Fiber is a type of carbohydrate that the body cannot digest (which is why it's sometimes called roughage). Because it is not digested, fiber passes through the digestive system intact. Fiber helps keep food moving through the digestive system, making the bowels more regular and preventing constipation. It can also help lower cholesterol and blood sugar levels to protect against the development of diseases such as diabetes. The best sources of fiber are fruits, vegetables, beans, and whole grains.

Magnesium

Magnesium, found in green leafy vegetables, almonds, and soybeans, is indispensable for so many of the body's functions that it would be impossible to mention all of its specific jobs in this chapter. About three hundred different chemical reactions in the body rely on magnesium. A few of magnesium's roles include keeping the heart rhythm steady and blood pressure normal, enabling nerves and muscles to function, supporting a healthy immune system, helping the body produce energy, and keeping the bones strong.

About half of the body's magnesium is found in the bones, and the rest is inside tissues and organs. Magnesium is stored in the intestines and transported to the cells and tissues through the bloodstream.

Fatty Acids

Not all fats are unhealthy. In fact, some are essential to the diet. Omega-3 fatty acids, found in nuts, seeds, and oils, keep the cells of

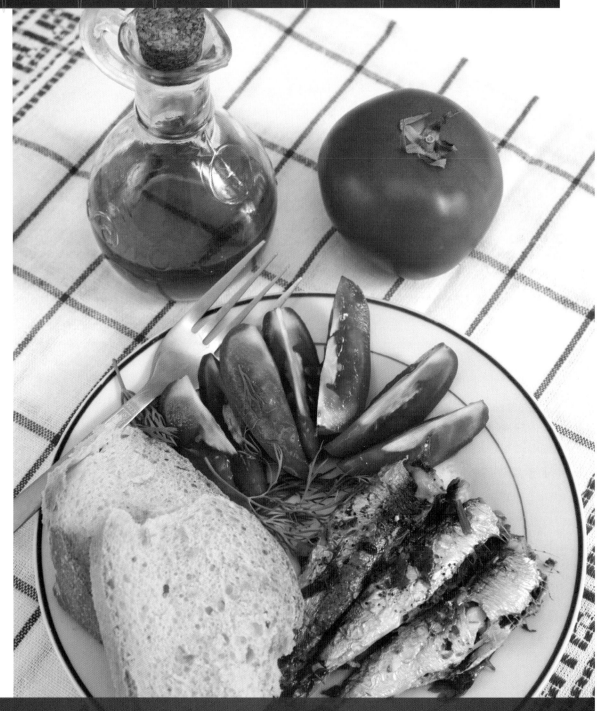

Sardines are high in omega-3 fatty acids, healthy fats that can help protect against heart disease. Salmon, mackerel, and trout are other good fish sources of omega-3 fatty acids.

the brain and nervous system functioning normally. Because the body cannot make these fatty acids, it is vital to get them through the diet.

Many researchers today have been investigating the ability of omega-3 fatty acids to prevent disease. They are finding that fatty acids reduce inflammation in the body and lower levels of cholesterol and triglycerides, reducing the risk for heart disease.

Fatty acids are especially important in babies, who are still developing. Infants need a type of fatty acid called docosahexaenoic acid (DHA), which is found in breast milk. DHA helps a baby's brain, nervous system, immune system, and vision develop.

Other Nutrients

Many more important components of a healthy diet exist than are described in this chapter. The following are just a few of the other nutrients people need on a regular basis:

- **Sodium:** Helps fluid move in and out of cells, and aids in muscle contraction and heart rhythm
- **Lycopene:** May protect against some forms of cancer
- **Chromium:** Is involved in regulating blood sugar
- **Selenium:** Helps the immune system fight infection and may protect against some forms of cancer
- **Silicon:** Keeps tissues strong to support healthy skin, hair, nails, joints, and connective tissues

People who don't eat a balanced diet may not get enough of these and other nutrients in their diet. Vitamin deficiencies can lead to some pretty serious diseases, which are described in the following chapter.

Ten Great Questions
to Ask a Health Professional

1 Can I get the vitamins and minerals I need daily from diet alone?

2 Do I need to take a multivitamin?

3 Do I have any health problems that affect my body's ability to absorb vitamins and minerals?

4 What vitamins and minerals are most important for me to get every day?

5 What kinds of foods should I be eating daily?

6 How can I buy supplements safely?

7 Do vitamins become more effective when I take more of them?

8 Can taking too much of certain vitamins be dangerous?

9 Do I need to take extra vitamins if I exercise?

10 Do my vitamin pills become ineffective after the expiration date?

Chapter 3

Dangers of Skimping on Vitamins and Minerals

Considering that people need vitamins and minerals to stay alive and remain healthy, it makes sense that not getting enough of these nutrients could lead to some serious health problems. A lack of enough vitamins or minerals is called a deficiency, and some deficiencies can be very dangerous.

Eating an unhealthy or limited diet is one way to become deficient in a nutrient. Someone who eats nothing but burgers, fries, and candy and washes these junk foods down with soft drinks will miss out on all the important vitamins and minerals contained in fruit, vegetables, dairy foods, and whole grains. Even though eating fruits and vegetables is generally healthy, vegetarians can lack enough protein and other nutrients found in meat if they don't eat the right kinds of vegetable-based foods or take a daily supplement.

Vitamin and mineral deficiencies can have other causes as well. Certain medications can prevent the body from properly absorbing vitamins or minerals, or they can cause the body to release too much of those nutrients in the urine. Health conditions such as Crohn's disease or celiac disease can prevent the intestines from properly absorbing vitamins or minerals. Growing older can affect both a person's diet and his or her likelihood of getting diseases that can interfere with vitamin and mineral absorption. As people age, they tend to eat

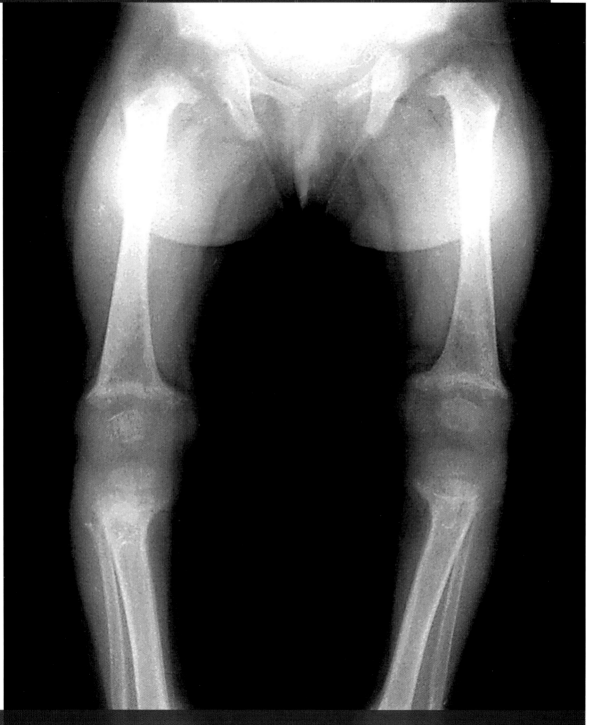

This X-ray shows the soft, deformed bones of a child with rickets. This disease is caused by a lack of vitamin D, calcium, or phosphorus.

less because they are not as hungry or they have difficulty preparing food for themselves, which also puts them at risk for deficiencies.

Vitamin and Mineral Deficiencies

Each of the vitamins and minerals listed in chapters 1 and 2 has an important purpose. The following are just some of the health problems that can occur in people who don't get enough of certain nutrients:

Vitamin A. A lack of vitamin A in the diet can lead to damage in the retina and cornea of the eye. Although vitamin A deficiency is rare in the United States, it is still common in other parts of the world, especially in poor nations. Between 250,000 and 500,000 children in

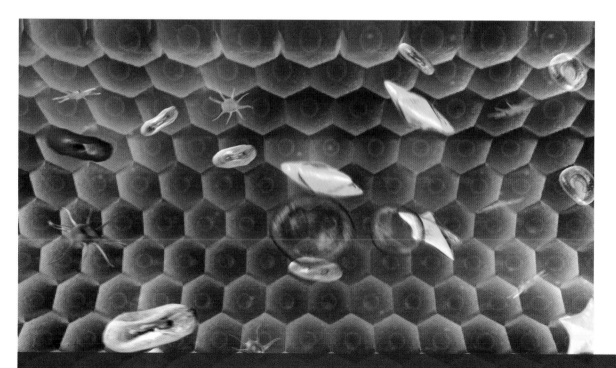

Homocysteine is an amino acid in the blood. A lack of B vitamins in the diet can raise homocysteine levels, which have been linked to a higher risk for heart disease.

developing countries become blind each year because they do not get enough vitamin A in their diet, according to the Office of Dietary Supplements at the National Institutes of Health. Vitamin A deficiency also makes it more difficult for the body to fight off infections.

Vitamin B. A lack of folic acid and other B vitamins can lead to high levels of an amino acid called homocysteine in the blood. Excess homocysteine can increase a person's risk for getting heart disease, as well as the brain disorder Alzheimer's disease. Folic acid deficiency is especially dangerous during pregnancy. Pregnant women who do not get enough folic acid can have a baby born prematurely, at low birth weight, or with a serious birth defect such as spina bifida.

Vitamin D. Adequate amounts of vitamin D are essential for maintaining levels of calcium and phosphorus in the blood. Without enough vitamin D, the bones can lose calcium and become weak and easily breakable. Vitamin D deficiency has also been linked to an increased risk for heart disease, diabetes, and cancer.

Vitamin K. The body needs vitamin K for the blood to clot. People who do not get enough of this vitamin may bleed or bruise easily.

Calcium. Calcium is crucial in keeping bones healthy. Some people have trouble eating dairy foods (which are high in calcium) because they are lactose intolerant. Their bodies cannot break down lactose, a sugar found in milk and other dairy products. Other people just don't like eating dairy products. Whatever the reason, when there is not enough calcium in the diet, the body has its own way of maintaining the balance. It pulls calcium out of the bones and moves it into the bloodstream. Removing calcium from the bones weakens them, increasing a person's risk of getting a nasty break or fracture. People who are calcium-deficient are also at risk for tooth decay and heart problems.

The deficiencies listed in this chapter are just a few of the problems that can occur from not getting enough vitamins and minerals. Several diseases are also linked to nutrient deficiencies.

Diseases Linked to Low Levels of Vitamins and Nutrients

The knowledge that a lack of certain vitamins and minerals can lead to disease isn't a new idea. Even the ancient Egyptians understood that people who did not eat enough liver were more likely to develop night blindness. Many centuries later, scientists discovered that liver is a rich source of vitamin A, which is important for eye health.

All of the following diseases have historically been linked to vitamin and mineral deficiencies:

Scurvy. Hundreds of years ago, sailors who traveled on ships for months or years often developed strange symptoms. Their skin became pale and covered with large spots, they were tired all of the time, and their teeth rotted and fell out. Eventually, many sailors died from this unknown affliction. In 1497, Portuguese navigator Vasco da Gama set sail from Lisbon, Portugal. He was headed around the Cape of Good Hope to establish a European trading colony on the coast of India. Da Gama left with a crew of 160 men. By the end of his voyage, he had lost one hundred of his sailors due to this strange illness.

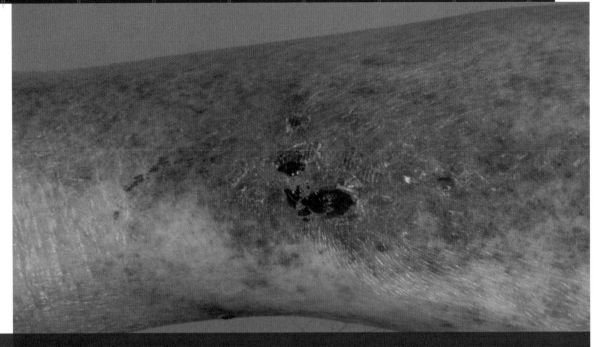

Scurvy is a disease caused by a lack of vitamin C. It weakens tiny blood vessels called capillaries, leading to bleeding in the skin.

In 1601, an explorer named Captain James Lancaster tested out a theory that citrus fruit might protect his crew against the illness that was killing so many sailors. On a voyage from England to India, he gave the men on one of his ships three teaspoons of lemon juice a day. The men on the other ships did not receive any juice. Halfway through the trip, 40 percent of the sailors on Lancaster's other ships had died. None of the sailors who took the lemon juice died.

It wasn't until 1746 that a British naval surgeon named James Lind established for certain that citrus fruits such as oranges and lemons, which are high in vitamin C, could prevent scurvy—the mysterious disease responsible for the deaths of so many sailors. Scurvy, or vitamin C deficiency, weakens the tiny blood vessels in the body called capillaries, causing the gums to bleed and the teeth to loosen.

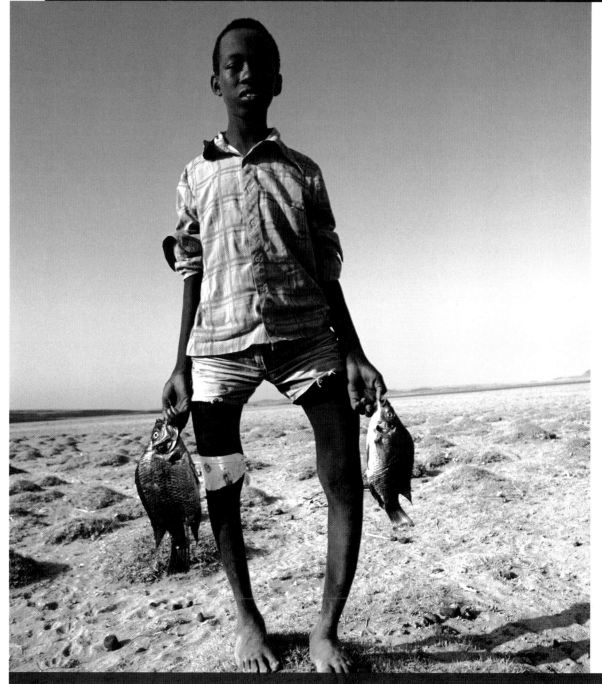

This child's legs are bent due to rickets, a disease caused by insufficient vitamin D in the diet or a lack of exposure to sunlight. Rickets causes the bones to become weak, soft, and deformed, especially in young people, when their skeletal bones are still growing.

Scurvy also prevents the body from making enough red blood cells, which are needed to transport oxygen to the organs and tissues (this is why sailors who had scurvy felt so tired all of the time). Eventually, citrus fruits became a staple on every ocean voyage, and scurvy stopped being a problem. Today, scurvy is rare, but it can still occur in people who do not get enough vitamin C in their diet.

Rickets. Children who don't get enough vitamin D in their diet or through sunlight can get a condition called rickets. This disease causes children's bones and teeth to become weak, and it can eventually leave children deformed. At the beginning of the twentieth century, many children living in poverty in the northern United States developed rickets.

By the 1930s, doctors had learned that taking cod liver oil could prevent rickets. For many years, parents gave their children this foul-tasting treatment every day to protect against the disease. Today, thanks to fortified dairy products and other foods, rickets is rare in the United States and children are no longer forced to endure cod liver oil every day. However, babies and toddlers can still be at risk for the disease if they don't get enough vitamin D because their bones are growing so quickly and use so much of the vitamin. Baby formula does contain vitamin D, but babies who are breast-fed may need to take a supplement (as is currently recommended by the American Academy of Pediatrics).

Beriberi. In 1630, Dutch doctor Jacobus Bontius discovered an unusual disease on the Indonesian island of Java. He noted that people with the disease walked like sheep with their knees shaking and their legs raised. The inhabitants of Java called the disease "beriberi," a name that means sheep.

Two forms of beriberi exist. The "wet form" affects the heart, causing increased heart rate and shortness of breath. The "dry form" affects the nervous system, leading to difficulty in walking and loss of feeling in parts of the body.

Doctors now know that beriberi is caused by a deficiency of thiamine (vitamin B_1). Beriberi is uncommon in the United States because many foods are enriched with thiamine. However, in rare cases, it can still occur in people who do not eat a healthy diet.

Pellagra. The word "pellagra" means "rough skin" in Italian. It describes one of the main symptoms of a lack of niacin (vitamin B_3). Niacin deficiency can damage not only the skin, but also almost every other organ in the body. Eventually, the disease can lead to death.

In the early 1900s, pellagra was common among poor people in the South, and doctors mistakenly believed that germs were responsible. In 1914, Joseph Goldberger, a doctor in the U.S. Public Health Service, traveled around the southern states researching pellagra. He discovered that diet was actually to blame for the disease. Southern farmers were not getting enough niacin in their diet because they ate almost nothing but corn. Today, many foods are fortified with niacin, so pellagra rarely occurs in the United States.

Anemia. A lack of iron or a deficiency of any of several B vitamins (vitamins B_6 and B_{12}) can lead to anemia. Iron deficiency is the single greatest nutritional problem in the world. It affects up to 80 percent of the world's population (four to five billion people), according to the Centers for Disease Control and Prevention. Young girls and women are at the greatest risk for anemia because they lose iron every month in their menstrual flow.

The Goiter Belt

A goiter is a condition in which the thyroid gland becomes enlarged. It occurs when the thyroid does not have the iodine it needs to produce enough of its hormones. In the early 1900s, an area of the United States that stretched across the Midwest and around the Great Lakes became known as the Goiter Belt. That name was given to the region because the soil in those areas was so lacking in iodine that large numbers of residents developed thyroid swelling. After doing some research, doctors discovered that adding iodine to salt in the diet could prevent these goiters. Thanks to the introduction of iodized salt in the 1920s, goiters have become far less common today.

People who have anemia lack enough red blood cells. These blood cells transport oxygen to the body's organs. As a result, people with this disease feel tired and weak, and they may have headaches. Children with chronic anemia may have more difficulty learning than their healthy peers.

Risks of Taking Too Much of Some Vitamins and Minerals

Vitamins and minerals are an important part of a healthy diet. However, just as a deficiency of certain nutrients can be harmful to one's health, taking too much of certain vitamins and minerals can also be danger-ous. This is especially true of fat-soluble vitamins, which are stored in the body instead of being eliminated by the kidneys.

The U.S. government has established tolerable upper intake levels (ULs) for vitamins and minerals. ULs refer to the maximum dose of a vitamin or mineral that a person can take before becoming sick. It is difficult to exceed the UL for any nutrient by eating large amounts of foods alone. However, taking megadoses (very high doses) of vitamins and minerals in supplement form can lead to dangerously high levels of these substances in the body.

The following are some of the side effects that can occur when people take too much of certain nutrients:

Vitamin A can be toxic in large amounts. Immediately after eating too much vitamin A, a person may feel dizzy and nauseated. He or she might vomit or have a severe headache. Side effects of vitamin A overdose include birth defects, liver problems, weakened bones, and disorders of the central nervous system. A person who eats a lot of carrots (which are high in vitamin A) usually won't have side effects, but the carrots might turn the person's skin orange.

The UL for vitamin A for teens is 1,700 to 2,800 micrograms per day.

Vitamin D affects calcium levels in the body. Taking too much of this vitamin may cause nausea, vomiting, weakness, or

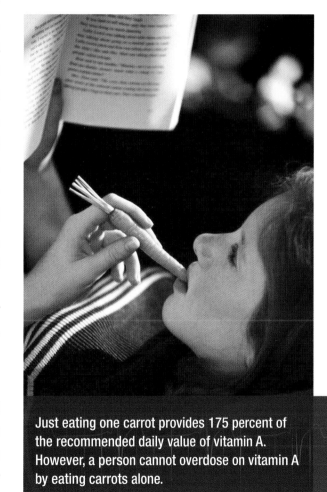

Just eating one carrot provides 175 percent of the recommended daily value of vitamin A. However, a person cannot overdose on vitamin A by eating carrots alone.

poor appetite. Excess vitamin D can cause levels of calcium in the blood to rise dangerously. High calcium levels can affect the brain and heart. The person may become confused or experience a change in heart rhythm. Excess vitamin D can also deposit in the kidneys, leading to painful masses called kidney stones. It's difficult to get too much vitamin D from exposure to the sun alone, but it is possible to get too much by overdosing on vitamin D supplements or taking more than the recommended daily dose of cod liver oil. The UL for vitamin D for teens is 50 micrograms per day.

B vitamins are water-soluble. When a person eats too much of these vitamins, his or her body generally flushes out the excess. However, there have been reported cases of people having side effects after taking large doses of some B vitamins. Taking large amounts of vitamin B_6 can damage the nerves in the arms and legs, causing people to lose feeling in those limbs. Vitamin B_3 overdose can cause redness of the skin and an upset stomach. Taking excess amounts of vitamin B_1 can lead to heart problems. The UL for vitamin B_1 for teens has not been established. The UL for vitamin B_3 is 20 to 30 milligrams per day, and the UL for vitamin B_6 is 60 to 80 milligrams per day.

Vitamin C in large doses has been linked to kidney stones and other kidney problems, although research has not confirmed this side effect. Some evidence exists that vitamin C can interfere with certain medications that people take, such as the blood thinner warfarin (brand name Coumadin). Vitamin C might also change the results of certain laboratory tests, making it difficult for the doctor to determine whether the test is positive or negative. The UL for vitamin C for teens is 1,200 to 1,800 milligrams per day.

Vitamin E has been linked to some pretty serious side effects. It can lead to excess bleeding, especially when people take it at the same time as blood-thinning medicines. There is even some evidence that people who take very high doses of vitamin E every day face a greater risk of dying than the general population. The UL for vitamin E for teens is 600 to 800 milligrams per day.

Calcium can build up in the blood. When blood that is too high in calcium reaches the kidneys to be filtered, it can damage the kidneys. Excess calcium can also interfere with the body's absorption of iron, magnesium, zinc, and phosphorus. Calcium supplements can interact with several different medicines, including heart drugs, antibiotics, seizure medications, and medicines given to treat the bone-thinning disease osteoporosis. The UL for calcium for teens is 2,500 milligrams per day.

Iron can be very dangerous when people take too much of it because the body removes very little iron in the urine. As a result, iron can quickly build up in the body's tissues and organs. Symptoms of iron overdose include upset stomach and constipation. Children have even died from accidental iron overdoses. The UL for iron for teens is 40 to 45 milligrams per day.

To avoid all of these harmful side effects, people should get their nutrients mainly through eating food, rather than taking supplements. People who have to take supplements because they are not getting enough vitamins and minerals from food alone should never take more than the daily DRI for their age and gender. It's important for people taking supplements to let their doctor know exactly what kind of supplement they are taking to avoid possible side effects or drug interactions.

MYTHS and FACTS

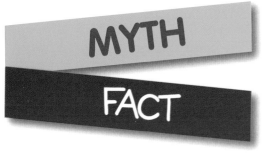

MYTH The more vitamins people take, the healthier they will become.

FACT The Institute of Medicine has established Dietary Reference Intakes (DRIs) describing how much of each vitamin and mineral people need each day. Each person's DRI differs depending on his or her age and gender. Taking more than the DRI of certain vitamins can be very dangerous. This is especially true for fat-soluble vitamins, which can build up in the body.

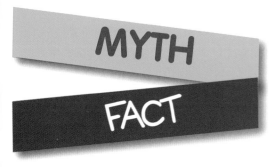

MYTH Vitamin and mineral supplements are perfectly safe because they are all natural.

FACT Just because something is labeled "all natural" doesn't mean that it's safe. Taking more than the recommended amount of any vitamin or mineral can be dangerous to one's health. Some vitamins can interact with medications, making them more or less potent. For example, vitamin

A can thin the blood. Taking vitamin A with medications that already thin the blood can cause a person to bleed excessively. Because of the potential for interactions, it's important for people to tell their doctor and pharmacist about every single medicine and supplement they are taking.

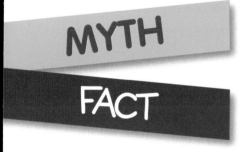

MYTH

If you take a multivitamin every day, you can eat whatever you want.

FACT

A multivitamin can enrich the diet, but it is no replacement for healthy eating. Natural foods contain a variety of nutrients that can never be captured in a bottle. Apples, for example, are packed with antioxidants, fiber, and vitamin C. A glass of fortified milk is high in both calcium and vitamin D. Eating many different types of fruits, vegetables, dairy products, whole grains, and lean meats is still the best and most efficient way to give the body the nutrition it needs.

Chapter 4

Building a Healthy, Balanced Diet

It is possible to get all of the vitamins and minerals a person needs to stay healthy just by eating three balanced meals every day. The trouble is, very few people actually eat the right kind of diet. More than 80 percent of Americans eat fewer than the recommended servings of fruit, vegetables, and whole grains, according to the U.S. Preventive Services Task Force. Most Americans also don't get enough calcium, iron, and fiber in their diet, says the U.S. Food and Drug Administration.

Poor eating habits are contributing to an epidemic of health problems. The Centers for Disease Control and Prevention report that more than two-thirds of people in this country are either overweight or obese, including nearly 20 percent of teens. More than twenty-three million Americans have diabetes, a disease that is often caused by being overweight or obese. Diabetes can lead to numerous health complications, including heart disease and kidney failure.

Eating the right foods, in the right amounts, can prevent obesity and ensure good health. Yet today, many people are busy and rely on convenience foods that contain very little nutrition. Knowing the elements of a balanced diet and planning meals ahead of time can help make it easier to eat healthily.

The Elements of a Healthy Diet

According to the U.S. Department of Agriculture's MyPyramid food guide, every diet should contain the following six elements:

1. **Grains:** 5 to 7 ounces (142 to 198 grams) each day of whole grains, including brown rice, oatmeal, whole-wheat bread, and popcorn. (One slice of whole-wheat bread or 1 cup [240 milliliters] of cereal equals 1 ounce [28 grams].)
2. **Vegetables:** 2 to 3 cups (470 to 710 ml) every day of different-colored vegetables, including broccoli, carrots, sweet potatoes,

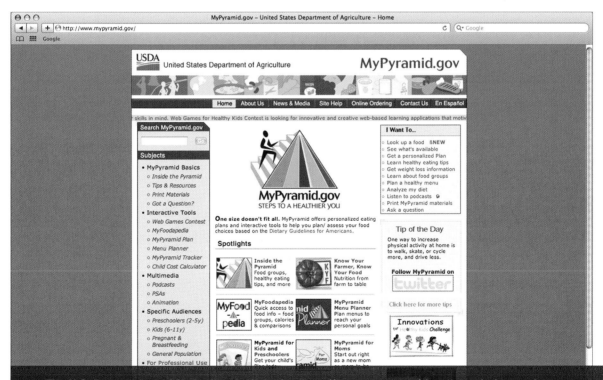

The U.S. Department of Agriculture's Web site (http://www.mypyramid.gov) can help people design personalized healthy eating plans based on their age, gender, and activity level.

corn, lima beans, and black-eyed peas. (One large sweet potato equals 1 cup [240 ml] of vegetables.)

3. **Fruits:** 1 ½ cups (350 ml) per day of a variety of fruits, including apples, oranges, cantaloupe, strawberries, blueberries, papaya, and nectarines.

4. **Milk:** 3 cups (710 ml) each day of low-fat or skim milk, cheese, and yogurt.

5. **Meat and beans:** 5 to 6 ounces (141 to 170 grams) every day of lean beef, chicken, turkey, fish, eggs, nuts, and beans.

6. **Oils:** 5 to 6 teaspoons (25 to 30 ml) per day of vegetable oil (canola, olive, safflower), nuts, oily fish, or avocados.

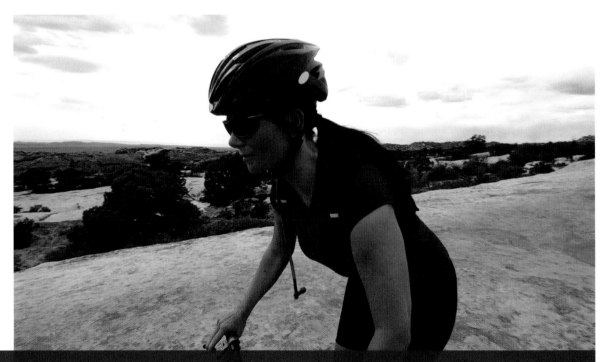

In addition to eating a well-balanced diet, the U.S. Department of Agriculture recommends that an individual get at least a half hour each day of moderate exercise, such as cycling, walking, dancing, or playing a sport.

A sample healthy menu might look something like the following, which has been adapted from the MyPyramid.gov recommendations:

- **Breakfast:** One whole-wheat English muffin with 2 teaspoons (10 ml) of soft margarine and 1 tablespoon (15 ml) of jam or preserves, one medium grapefruit, one hard-boiled egg, and one unsweetened drink
- **Lunch:** Tuna fish sandwich on rye bread with 2 teaspoons (10 ml) of mayonnaise and two slices of tomato, one medium pear, one cup (240 ml) of fat-free milk
- **Dinner:** 3 ounces (85 grams) of roasted, boneless, skinless chicken breast; one large baked sweet potato; ½ cup (120 ml) of peas and onions with 1 teaspoon (5 ml) of soft margarine; one whole-wheat dinner roll (1 ounce [24 grams]) with one teaspoon (5 ml) of soft margarine; and 1 cup (240 ml) of leafy greens salad with 3 teaspoons (15 ml) of sunflower oil and vinegar dressing
- **Snacks:** 1 cup (240 ml) of low-fat fruit yogurt

Add to this healthy diet plan a generous dose of exercise. Aim for at least thirty minutes of moderate-to-vigorous walking, dancing, swimming, bicycling, aerobics, or sports each day.

Superfoods and Superduds

There is a reason why nutrition experts are always pushing fruits and vegetables as part of a healthy diet. Many of these foods are packed with natural substances such as antioxidants, which can actually fight off disease. The following are just a few of these "superfoods":

- **Carrots:** Contain carotenoids, which help protect the eyes from cataracts and macular degeneration.
- **Spinach:** Rich in folic acid, which can help prevent birth defects, and vitamin K, which helps the blood clot.
- **Apples:** The skin is high in fiber, which can help keep the digestive system regular.
- **Blueberries:** High in antioxidants, which may protect against cancer and Alzheimer's disease.
- **Cranberries:** Help prevent urinary tract infections and contain antioxidants that may lower the risk of heart disease or stroke.

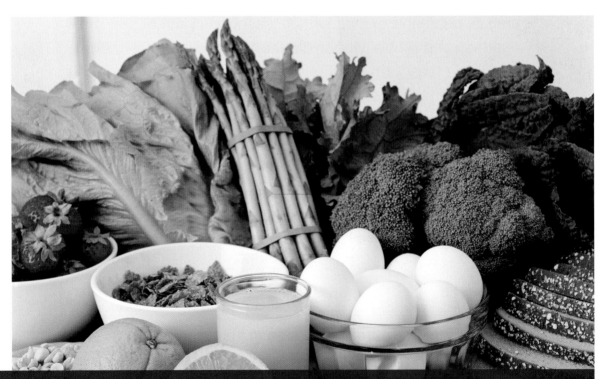

Superfoods such as broccoli, asparagus, strawberries, nuts, and spinach are filled with a variety of nutrients and antioxidants that can help protect against disease.

- **Grapes:** The skin contains resveratrol, which boosts levels of "good" HDL cholesterol and protects the heart.
- **Broccoli and beets:** Contain natural substances called flavonoids that may help ward off cancer.
- **Flaxseed and fatty fish (such as tuna):** High in omega-3 fatty acids, which can protect the heart and brain from disease.

The "superduds" of the diet are those foods that are high in fat and calories and low in nutrients. Superduds include fried foods (French fries), highly processed foods, fast food, and soda pops. Filling up on nutrient-rich superfoods will leave less room in the diet for superduds like sweets and high-fat foods.

Food Sources of Important Vitamins and Minerals

The list below includes many of the foods that are high in each important vitamin and mineral. Everyone should try to include a combination of these foods in their daily diet:

- **Vitamin A:** Carrots, sweet potatoes, mangoes, cantaloupes, apricots, spinach, kale, liver, eggs, fatty fish (salmon, herring, some tuna), fortified breakfast cereals, and milk and other dairy products
- **Vitamin B$_1$:** Brown rice, oatmeal, dried beans, chicken, fish, liver, sunflower seeds, beans, and enriched whole-grain bread
- **Vitamin B$_2$:** Dairy products, eggs, green leafy vegetables, nuts, chicken, salmon, whole-grain breads and cereals, almonds, and avocados

- **Vitamin B$_3$:** Peanuts and peanut butter, tuna, mackerel, liver, eggs, chicken, whole grains, avocados, dried fruits, and fortified cereals
- **Vitamin B$_5$:** Milk, beef liver, trout, broccoli, dried beans, peas, mushrooms, cashews, brown rice, and oats
- **Vitamin B$_6$:** Chicken, fish, pork, beef, nuts, beans, eggs, bananas, avocados, and fortified cereals
- **Vitamin B$_8$:** Liver, kidney, egg yolks, rice, yeast, and soybeans
- **Folic acid:** Leafy green vegetables (spinach, turnip greens, kale), fruits (oranges and orange juice, papaya), dried beans and peas, fortified breads and cereals, and peanuts
- **Vitamin B$_{12}$:** Clams, liver, trout, beef, salmon, sardines, mackerel, yogurt, milk, cheese, fortified breakfast cereals, and egg yolk
- **Vitamin C:** Oranges, lemons, tangerines, grapefruit, papaya, melon, broccoli, Brussels sprouts, collard greens, and sweet peppers
- **Vitamin D:** Milk and other fortified dairy products, salmon, mackerel, sardines, fortified cereal, and eggs
- **Vitamin E:** Wheat germ oil, sunflower seeds and oil, almonds, peanuts and peanut butter, spinach, broccoli, butter, green leafy vegetables, wheat germ, and whole grains
- **Vitamin K:** Leafy green vegetables (spinach, cabbage, turnip greens, lettuce), yogurt, eggs, and soybean and canola oils
- **Calcium:** Milk, cheese, yogurt, almonds, apricots, beans, broccoli, mustard and collard greens, salmon, sardines with bones, tofu, and kale
- **Iodine:** Cabbage, kale, Brussels sprouts, cauliflower, shellfish, meats, eggs, whole grains, salt, nuts, and seeds

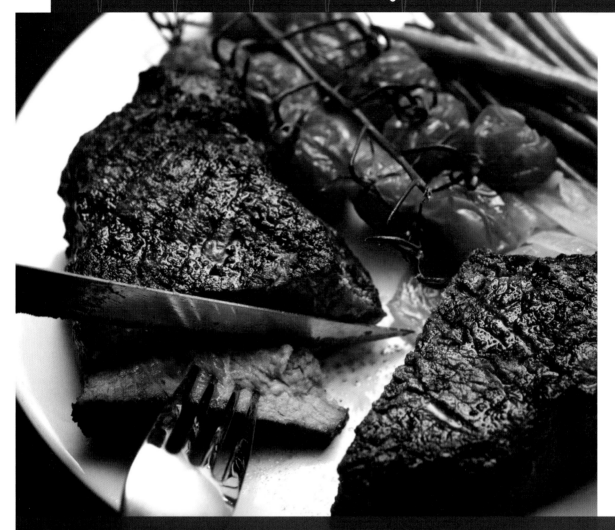

Red meat can be part of a healthy diet, but only in moderation. The U.S. Department of Agriculture recommends that teens eat just 5 to 6 ounces (142 to 170 grams) of lean red meat each day.

- **Iron:** Beef, chicken, oysters, clams, tuna, liver, fortified cereal, soybeans, lentils, tofu, spinach, nuts, seeds, raisins, and prunes
- **Magnesium:** Spinach, beans and peas, nuts and seeds, wheat flour, halibut, peanuts, almonds, cashews, soybeans, baked potato (skin on), soybeans, lentils, and sunflower seeds

- **Potassium:** Butternut squash, bananas, lima beans, pinto beans, papaya, cantaloupe, avocado, raisins, chard, dates, nuts and seeds, whole grains, and apricots
- **Phosphorus:** Liver, cheese, whole-wheat bread, lean beef, eggs, milk, corn, oatmeal, green beans, broccoli, oranges, nuts, and seeds
- **Zinc:** Oysters, beef, pork, fortified cereal, chicken, baked beans, chickpeas, cashews, yogurt, cheese, and milk
- **Omega-3 fatty acids:** Cold-water fish (salmon, tuna, mackerel, sardines, trout), nuts, seeds, and vegetable oils

"Variety is the spice of life," as the old saying goes. Variety is also key to a healthy diet. Eating a lot of different fruits, vegetables, whole grains, dairy products, and meats will ensure that people get all of the vitamins and minerals that they need to stay healthy.

How to Buy a Vitamin or Nutritional Supplement

When buying any vitamin or mineral supplement, it's important to read the label carefully. Products should contain no more than 100 percent of the Recommended Dietary Intake of each vitamin and mineral for the person's age. Look for the letters "USP" on the label. This means that the supplement meets the standards set by the U.S. Pharmacopeia, a public health organization, for strength and purity.

Finally, people should be careful not to believe the supplement industry hype. If a bottle reads "all natural" or "cures disease," it may not be true. It's important to always check with a doctor before buying any supplement.

Multivitamins and Supplements: Balanced Nutrition in a Pill?

Supplements have become a big business in the United States. Americans spend almost $2 billion on different vitamin and mineral supplements each year. One study in the February 2009 edition of the *Archives of Pediatrics and Adolescent Medicine* found that more than one-third of children had taken a vitamin and/or mineral supplement in the past month.

Yet health experts say teens who eat a balanced, nutritious diet may not need additional vitamins or minerals. In fact, the American Academy of Pediatrics does not recommend supplemental vitamins for most healthy children over the age of one. However, picky or limited eaters or those with special health concerns may benefit from a nutritional supplement. The following are a few reasons why some people might need to take a daily vitamin or mineral supplement:

- They eat a poor diet that does not include a variety of fruits, vegetables, whole grains, dairy products, and meats.
- They eat a vegetarian or vegan (no animal or dairy products) diet, and don't get enough of vitamin B_{12} or other important nutrients.
- They are pregnant or breastfeeding and need extra vitamins and minerals to support the baby's nutritional needs.
- They have a medical condition that affects their diet or their body's absorption of nutrients (such as a food allergy or intestinal disease).

Supplements come in many different forms: chewables, tablets, capsules, liquids, and even gummy bears (children need to be careful

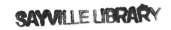

not to eat more than the daily dosage of these candylike vitamins). Because the U.S. Food and Drug Administration does not regulate supplements, it's often difficult to know exactly what is in the bottle or whether that supplement is safe and effective. That is why it's very important to be a careful consumer when shopping for vitamin and mineral supplements.

Sneaking Vitamins and Minerals into the Diet

Even the pickiest of eaters can find ways to build a varied, healthy diet that contains all of the major food groups. There are a few tricks for sneaking foods into the diet that taste so good, a picky eater won't even realize that he or she is eating a healthy meal.

First, it helps to wait to eat until a person is hungry. This technique will not only prevent unhealthy snacking between meals, but it will also make everything on the plate suddenly seem more appealing. Second, try some tricks to make healthy food look and taste like fast food. Create sweet potato fries by cutting sweet potatoes into strips and baking them in the oven. Another method is to hide applesauce, oats, and even spinach inside chocolate brownies.

The key is to make everything in the diet delicious and appealing. People who love what they're eating will never miss junk food and soft drinks. Moreover, they will never have to worry that they are cheating themselves out of the nutrients they need to stay healthy.

age-related macular degeneration A disease that affects the retina in the eye, leading to a loss of central vision.

Alzheimer's disease A disease that affects people's memory and ability to care for themselves.

anemia A disease that reduces the number of red blood cells in the body. Red blood cells transport oxygen to the body's tissues.

antioxidants Vitamins and minerals that protect the body from damage caused by free radicals.

carotenoids Red, orange, and yellow color pigments found in many plants.

celiac disease A disease that affects the intestines and makes a person unable to eat gluten, a protein found in wheat.

cleft palate A birth defect that occurs when the roof of the mouth does not properly close during an infant's development. Taking folic acid during pregnancy can reduce the risk for this and other birth defects.

Crohn's disease A condition that affects the intestines, leading to cramps, diarrhea, and excessive weight loss. Crohn's disease can affect the body's ability to absorb certain nutrients.

deficiency A lack of one or more nutrients in the diet.

electrolytes Substances in the body, including sodium and potassium, that can conduct electric currents and help regulate cells' metabolism.

fat-soluble vitamins Vitamins such as A, D, E, and K that the body stores instead of removing in the urine.

free radicals Unstable molecules that can damage cells and possibly lead to changes that cause cancer.

goiter A condition in which the thyroid gland is enlarged. It is usually due to a lack of iodine in the diet.

hemoglobin The substance in red blood cells that transports oxygen to the body's tissues and organs.

high-density lipoprotein (HDL) cholesterol The "good" form of cholesterol that helps keep the arteries clear.

homocysteine An amino acid that is found in the blood. High levels of homocysteine have been linked to an increased risk for heart disease and blood clots.

lactose intolerance The inability to digest lactose, the sugar found in milk. People who are lactose intolerant become sick when they drink milk or eat foods that are made with milk.

low-density lipoprotein (LDL) cholesterol The "bad" form of cholesterol that can clog arteries and contribute to heart disease.

metabolism The processes by which the body's cells turn food into energy.

osteoporosis A disease in which the bones become thin and fragile and can break easily.

scurvy A disease caused by a deficiency in vitamin C, which can result in bleeding in the skin and gums.

spina bifida A birth defect in which an embryo's spine does not close correctly. Taking folic acid before and during pregnancy can help prevent this and other birth defects.

stroke The blockage of a blood vessel in the brain, which can lead to paralysis or even death.

water-soluble vitamins Vitamins that the body does not store, but removes in the urine. The B vitamins and vitamin C are examples of water-soluble vitamins.

American College of Nutrition
300 South Duncan Avenue, Suite 225
Clearwater, FL 33755
(727) 446-6086
Web site: http://www.americancollegeofnutrition.org
The goal of this organization is to promote education about proper
nutrition.

American Dietetic Association (ADA)
120 South Riverside Plaza, Suite 2000
Chicago, IL 60606-6995
(800) 877-1600
Web site: http://www.eatright.org
The biggest organization of dietitians in the world, the ADA provides
advice on healthy eating.

American Society for Nutrition
9650 Rockville Pike
Bethesda, MD 20814
(301) 634-7050
Web site: http://www.nutrition.org
The American Society for Nutrition brings together the top researchers
to advance the science of better nutrition.

Canadian Council of Food and Nutrition
2810 Matheson Boulevard East, 1st Floor
Mississauga, ON L4W 4X7
Canada

(905) 625-5746

Web site: http://www.ccfn.ca

This organization helps Canadians gain a better understanding of food and nutrition issues.

Dietitians of Canada

480 University Avenue, Suite 604

Toronto, ON M5G 1V2

Canada

(416) 596-0857

Web site: http://www.dietitians.ca

This organization is made up of dietitians who promote better health through diet to the people of Canada.

Healthy Kids Challenge

2 W Road 210

Dighton, KS 67839

(888) 259-6287

Web site: http://www.healthykidschallenge.com

This dietitian-led organization helps schools and communities take action to encourage young people to eat healthy foods and to get exercise.

U.S. Department of Agriculture (USDA)

1400 Independence Avenue SW

Washington, DC 20250

(202) 720-2791

Web site: http://www.usda.gov

The USDA has several programs, including MyPyramid, that promote healthy eating, exercise, and other lifestyle habits.

U.S. Food and Drug Administration (FDA)

10903 New Hampshire Avenue

Silver Spring, MD 20993-0002

(888) 463-6332

Web site: http://www.fda.gov

The FDA is the government organization that ensures that food, drugs, and supplements are safe for the American public.

Web Sites

Due to the changing nature of Internet links, Rosen Publishing has developed an online list of Web sites related to the subject of this book. This site is updated regularly. Please use this link to access the list:

http://www.rosenlinks.com/hab/vita

FOR FURTHER READING

Allred, Alexandra Powe. *Nutrition* (Reading Essentials in Science). Logan, IA: Perfection Learning, 2005.

Bickerstaff, Linda. *Nutrition Sense: Counting Calories, Figuring Out Fats, and Eating Balanced Meals* (Library of Nutrition). New York, NY: Rosen Publishing Group, 2004.

Claybourne, Anna. *Healthy Eating: Diet and Nutrition.* Portsmouth, NH: Heinemann, 2008.

Doeden, Matt. *Eat Right! How You Can Make Good Food Choices* (Health Zone). Minneapolis, MN: Lerner Publishing Group, 2009.

Douglas, Ann, and Julie Douglas. *Body Talk: The Straight Facts on Fitness, Nutrition, and Feeling Great About Yourself!* Toronto, ON: Maple Tree Press, 2006.

Dru Tecco, Betsy. *Food for Fuel* (Library of Nutrition). New York, NY: Rosen Publishing Group, 2008.

Faiella, Graham. *The Food Pyramid and Basic Nutrition: Assembling the Building Blocks of a Healthy Diet* (Library of Nutrition). New York, NY: Rosen Publishing Group, 2004.

Giddens, Sandra. *Making Smart Choices About Food, Nutrition, and Lifestyle.* New York, NY: Rosen Publishing Group, 2008.

Green, Emily K. *Meat and Beans* (New Food Guide Pyramid). Minneapolis, MN: Bellwether Media, 2006.

Harmon, Daniel E. *Obesity* (Coping in a Changing World). New York, NY: Rosen Publishing Group, 2007.

Johanson, Paula. *Processed Food* (What's in Your Food? Recipe for Disaster). New York, NY: Rosen Publishing Group, 2008.

Jukes, Mavis. *Be Healthy! It's a Girl Thing: Food, Fitness, and Feeling Great.* New York, NY: Crown Publishers, 2003.

Kainins, Daina. *YUM: Your Ultimate Manual for Good Nutrition.* Montreal, QC, Canada: Lobster Press, 2008.

Knighton, Kate. *Why Shouldn't I Eat Junk Food?* Eveleth, MN: Usborne Books, 2008.

McCarthy, Rose. *Food Labels* (Library of Nutrition). New York, NY: Rosen Publishing Group, 2008.

Peters, Celeste A. *Food* (Science Q&A). New York, NY: Weigl Publishers, 2009.

Royston, Angela. *Vitamins & Minerals for a Healthy Body.* Portsmouth, NH: Heinemann, 2009.

Sertori, Trisha. *Minerals and Vitamins.* South Yarra, VIC, Australia: Macmillan Publishers Australia, 2008.

Silate, Jennifer. *Planning and Preparing Healthy Meals and Snacks* (Library of Nutrition). New York, NY: Rosen Publishing Group, 2008.

Watson, Stephanie. *Trans Fats* (What's in Your Food? Recipe for Disaster). New York, NY: Rosen Publishing Group, 2008.

Wilson, Michael R. *Frequently Asked Questions About Staying Fit* (FAQ: Teen Life). New York, NY: Rosen Publishing Group, 2008.

BIBLIOGRAPHY

Centers for Disease Control and Prevention. "Micronutrient Facts." Retrieved September 23, 2009 (http://www.cdc.gov/immpact/micronutrients/index.html).

Centers for Disease Control and Prevention. "Obesity and Overweight." Retrieved September 26, 2009 (http://www.cdc.gov/nchs/fastats/overwt.htm).

GirlsHealth.gov. "Vitamins and Minerals." Retrieved August 22, 2009 (http://www.girlshealth.ogv/nutrition/essentials/index.cfm).

HealthDay. "Many Kids Don't Need the Vitamins They're Taking." February 2, 2009. Retrieved August 22, 2009 (http://health.usnews.com/articles/health/healthday/2009/02/02/many-kids-dont-need-the-vitamins-theyre-taking.html).

HealthDay. "Vitamin D Deficiency Linked to Heart Risk Factors in Kids." August 3, 2009. Retrieved August 22, 2009 (http://www.nlm.nih.gov/medlineplus/print/news/fullstory_87665.html).

Institute of Medicine. "Dietary Reference Intakes: Vitamins." Retrieved September 3, 2009 (http://www.iom.edu/Object.File/Master/7/296/webtablevitamins.pdf).

Khalsa, Dharma Singh. *Food as Medicine.* New York, NY: Atria Books, 2003.

Mann, Denise. "Vitamin D Deficiency Common in U.S. Children." CNN.com, August 3, 2009. Retrieved September 16, 2009 (http://www.cnn.com/2009/HEALTH/08/03/vitamin.d.children).

Mayo Clinic. "Dietary Supplements: Nutrition in a Pill?" Retrieved August 22, 2009 (http://www.mayoclinic.com/print/supplements/NU00198/METHOD=print).

Moreno, Megan A. "Vitamin and Mineral Supplementation in Children." *Archives of Pediatrics and Adolescent Medicine*, February 2009, Vol. 163, No. 2.

National Institutes of Health. "Dietary Supplement Fact Sheet: Calcium." Office of Dietary Supplements. Retrieved August 23, 2009 (http://ods.od.nih.gov/factsheets/calcium.asp).

National Institutes of Health. "Dietary Supplement Fact Sheet: Iron." Office of Dietary Supplements. Retrieved August 23, 2009 (http://ods.od.nih.gov/factsheets/iron.asp).

National Institutes of Health. "Dietary Supplement Fact Sheet: Vitamin A and Carotenoids." Office of Dietary Supplements. Retrieved August 23, 2009 (http://ods.od.nih.gov/factsheets/vitamina.asp).

National Institutes of Health. "Dietary Supplement Fact Sheet: Vitamin D." Office of Dietary Supplements. Retrieved August 23, 2009 (http://ods.od.nih.gov/factsheets/vitamind.asp).

U.S. Department of Agriculture. "Sample Menu at 2,000 Calorie Level." MyPyramid.gov. Retrieved September 27, 2009 (http://www.mypyramid.gov/tips_resources/menus.html).

U.S. Food and Drug Administration. "Fortify Your Knowledge About Vitamins." Retrieved August 22, 2009 (http://www.fda.gov/forconsumers/consumerupdates/ucm118079.htm).

U.S. Food and Drug Administration. "How to Understand and Use the Nutrition Facts Label." Retrieved September 27, 2009 (http://www.fda.gov/Food/LabelingNutrition/ConsumerInformation/ucm078889.htm).

U.S. Preventive Services Task Force. "Behavioral Counseling in Primary Care to Promote a Healthy Diet." Retrieved September 27, 2009 (http://www.ahrq.gov/clinic/3rduspstf/diet/dietrr.htm).

INDEX

A

Alzheimer's disease, 13, 30, 46
American Academy of Pediatrics, 34, 51
anemia, 35–36
antioxidants, 10, 13, 41, 45, 46

B

beriberi, 34–35
birth defects, 18, 30, 37
Bontius, Jacobus, 34
B vitamins, 4, 7, 14, 15–18, 30, 35, 38,
    47–48, 51

C

calcium, 4, 12–13, 14, 15, 19, 30–31, 38,
    41, 42, 48
cancer, 6, 10, 11, 12, 13, 25, 30, 46, 47
celiac disease, 27
Centers for Disease Control and
    Prevention, 35, 42
Crohn's disease, 27

D

diabetes, 6, 23, 30, 42
diet, building a balanced, 4, 6, 42–52
Dietary Reference Intakes (DRIs), 14,
    39, 40

E

electrolytes, 22
exercise, 6, 26, 45

F

fat-soluble vitamins, 7, 9, 36, 40
fiber, 23, 41, 42, 46

folic acid, 18, 30, 46, 48
free radicals, 10

G

Da Gama, Vasco, 31
goiter, 36
Goldberger, Joseph, 35

H

health professional, ten great questions to
    ask a, 26
heart disease, 6, 13, 16, 18, 25, 30, 42, 46
high-density lipoprotein (HDL), 16, 47

I

immune system, 4, 9, 13, 16, 22, 23, 25
Institute of Medicine, 14, 40
iodine, 22, 36, 48
iron, 4, 11, 14, 21, 22, 35, 38, 39, 42, 49

K

kidney stones, 38

L

lactose intolerance, 30
Lancaster, James, 32
Lind, James, 32
low-density lipoprotein (LDL), 16

M

macular degeneration, 13, 46
magnesium, 4, 14, 23, 39, 49
metabolism, 15, 16, 22
multivitamins, 26, 41
MyPyramid, 43, 45

N

National Institutes of Health, 30
night blindness, 31

O

obesity, 6, 42
Office of Dietary Supplements, 30
omega-3 fatty acids, 23, 25, 47, 50
osteoporosis, 15, 39

P

Pauling, Linus, 11
pellagra, 35
phosphorus, 13, 22, 30, 39, 50
potassium, 4, 14, 21–22, 50

R

Recommended Daily Allowance (RDA), 14
rickets, 34

S

salt/sodium, 6, 22, 25, 36
scurvy, 31–32, 34
supplements, 11, 12, 26, 37, 39, 40–41, 50, 51–52
Szent-Györgyi, Albert, 10

U

upper intake levels (ULs), 36–37, 38, 39
U.S. Department of Agriculture, 43

U.S. Food and Drug Administration, 42, 52
U.S. Pharmacopeia, 50
U.S. Preventative Services Task Force, 42
U.S. Public Health Service, 35

V

vegans, 51
vegetarians, 27, 51
vitamin A, 4, 7, 9–10, 14, 29–30, 37, 41, 47
vitamin C, 4, 7, 10–11, 14, 32, 34, 38, 41, 48
vitamin D, 4, 6, 7, 11–13, 14, 19, 30, 34, 37–38, 41, 48
vitamin E, 4, 7, 13, 14, 38, 48
vitamin K, 4, 7, 13, 14, 15, 30, 46, 48
vitamins and minerals,
    dangers of skimping on, 6, 25, 27–39
    myths and facts about, 40–41
    and other essential ingredients for a healthy diet, 19–25
    an overview of, 4–18

W

water-soluble vitamins, 7, 9, 15, 38

Z

zinc, 4, 22, 39, 50

About the Author

Stephanie Watson is an award-winning health and science writer based in Atlanta, Georgia. She is a regular contributor to several online and print publications, and she has written or contributed to more than two dozen books, including *Fast Food*, *Trans Fats*, and *This Is Me: Facing Physical Challenges.*

Photo Credits

Designer: Nicole Russo; Editor: Kathy Kuhtz Campbell;
Photo Researcher: Marty Levick